I0136071

Dash Diet

The Definitive Guide To Healthful And Delicious Recipes
For Managing And Lowering Blood Pressure

*(Recipes And Exercise Routines For Lowering Blood
Pressure And Enhancing Your Health)*

Christophe McGowan

TABLE OF CONTENT

Introduction

The original research led to the development of a healthy nutrition plan known as the Dash Diet, which assisted individuals in lowering their blood pressure, also known as hypertension.

In addition, researchers from various institutions concluded that the Dash diet is one of the best diets to implement if you suffer from one of the four conditions.,

This book will explain how the Dash Diet works and how you and your family can adhere to this multifaceted eating plan. In the first section, we will discuss the history and purpose of the DASH diet. The second section provides in-depth information about the benefits and complexities of the Dash Diet, including a nutrition chart broken down and explained in straightforward language. In Chapters III and IV, I will provide you with easy-to-prepare recipes for breakfast, lunch, and dinner, as well as nibbles and beverages that will provide you with energy throughout the day.

Here is my book, Dash Diet: The 2-Week Diet Plan for Weight Loss, so that you no longer have to fret about your life's longevity and lifestyle fluctuations – Your comprehensive guide to a healthful lifestyle.

DASH Diet Sodium Study

One of the key components of the DASH diet is a reduction in daily sodium intake. The purpose of the initial study was to determine whether a lower sodium injust take could improve the effectiveness of hypertension treatment. The researchers were inquisitive about the precise effects of sodium on the human body in comparison to a simple diet consisting of eating more fruits and vegetables.

When participants were given one of the two regimens, there were three distinct sodium concentrations. One contains 6 ,000 mg, while the other contains 2,8 00 mg and 2 ,10 00 mg. Thirty days of monitoring were performed on the participants. At the conclusion of the study, it was determined that a reduction in sodium injust take resulted in substantially lower diastolic and systolic blood pressure in both the DASH and control diet groups. The results led the researchers to conclude that the U.S. Dietary Guidelines for the average American should ideally be lower than 2,6 00 mg of sodium per day. Therefore, it is recommended that adults with high blood pressure consume 2 ,10 00 mg or less of sodium per day.

Modern Day DASH Diet

Today, the DASH diet is incredibly straightforward to adhere to. Major emphasis is placed on the foods that you are already advised to consume. You will consume more fruits and vegetables, something we have taught you since you were in elementary school. In addition, the diet will include many nutrients from lean proteins, low-fat dairy products, and whole grains. The objective is to consume more fiber, protein, potassium, and calcium to provide your body with the nutrients it requires to really become and remain healthy! With the nutrients, you should also limit your sodium injust take to approximately 2 ,10 00 milligrams per day.

In comparison to forty other diets evaluated by a panel of health professionals, the DASH diet was ranked as the best overall diet. The U.S. news assigned it an overall score of 8 .2 in categories such as short-term usage, long-term usage, ease of following the diet, and the diet's overall healthiness.

This is a remarkable accomplishment, but the diet also appeared on other lists, including the second best diabetes diet, the first best healthy eating diet, the first best heart health diet, and the sixth best weight loss diet.

Ultimately, the DASH diet is about striking an equilibrium so that you can adhere to it over the long term. This is not intended to be a regimen that you follow for a few months and then abandon. The DASH diet will consist of foods that easy make you feel better while also being delicious. If this is not enough to persuade you, in the next chapter, we will discuss all of the incredible benefits that the DASH diet can bring to your life and hopefully improve it.

Chapter 1: Utilizing The Two-Phase Dash Diet To Promote Weight Loss

The DASH diet is not necessarily intended for weight loss. However, as you progress, it is likely that you will lose unwanted weight because the diet will help you easy make healthier food choices. Typically, the diet consists of approximately 2,000 calories per day. If you wish to lose weight, you may be required to consume fewer calories. You may also need to modify your portion sizes based on your circumstances.

Typically, foods on the DASH diet are minimal in sodium. Some strategies to reduce sodium consumption include:

Not adding salt to hot cereal, pasta, or rice while preparing.

Substituting sodium-free flavorings or spices for salt in culinary preparation.

Purchasing foods labeled as'sodium-free,' 'low sodium,' 'no salt added,' or'very low sodium.'

Rinsing tinned foods to remove sodium.

Salt contains 2,6 210 milligrams of sodium per teaspoon. On food labels, certain processed foods contain excessive levels of sodium. Also high in sodium are low-fat canned vegetables, soups, sliced poultry, and ready-to-eat cereals.

When switching to the DASH diet, you may experience a change in flavor when consuming low-sodium beverages and foods. If your food tastes bland, progressively incorporate low-sodium foods and eliminate table salt until you reach your sodium goal. Utilizing salt-free seasoning herbs and mixtures can aid in the adjustment period. It may just take several weeks to wean yourself off of salted foods.

When adopting the DASH diet for improved health and weight loss, you may wish to adhere to the diet's two phases. After completing the two phases, a lifetime maintenance plan may be implemented.

During the first phase, which lasts approximately two weeks, you do not consume milk, cereals, or fruit, and you may only consume foods with very low starch content. In the second phase, designed for weight loss, you reintroduce milk, cereals, and fruit into your diet. During the phase of perpetual maintenance, you adhere to the second phase and indulge in occasional splurges.

Consult your dietitian or physician before adopting the DASH diet if you are diabetic and receiving treatment for your condition. The diet regimen can significantly reduce diabetes medication requirements. Therefore, you should not alter your medication without consulting your physician.

Step One

The first phase of the DASH Diet Weight Loss Solution consists of a two-week transition period designed to reset your metabolism. The protein-rich diet can help you lose weight quickly and just keep you feeling satisfied for longer.

Your liver, pancreas, and digestive hormones are given a rest from their normal intake.

By eliminating sugary and starchy foods from your diet, you prevent blood sugar increases. You will also avoid the constant lows and highs associated with most eating regimens.

First Phase Suggested Meal Planning

Consume protein at every meal and lunch

Here are some breakfast recommendations

V8 juice or tomato juice, if desired

2 -2 slices of Canadian prosciutto or bacon, or soy-free alternatives

yogurt artificially sweetened

Roll-ups of lean roast beef, poultry, ham, and low-fat cheese, and/or a lettuce wrap.

Fresh egg substitutes. However, you may consume fresh eggs with a small amount of cheese for the first 2 -2 days of mid-morning snacks. Consume at least two of the following recommendations.

Radishes, celery, cucumbers, carrots, cherry or grape tomatoes, and sliced red bell peppers.

Four ounces of low-fat cheese or mild cottage cheese.

Nuts (up to 2 /8 cup). If you consume cheese and almonds for lunch, limit nuts to one tablespoon. Choose a protein-rich main dish. You may also enjoy the following side dishes:

Jell-O (without sugar).

Vegetables and/or side salad

Tomatoes stuffed with fresh egg white salad, fresh egg salad, tuna salad, or chicken salad

Lean roast beef, turkey, or prosciutto rolled with low-fat cheese and/or a lettuce wrap.

Salad containing a variety of protein sources and vegetables, but no croutons. You can occasionally consume conventional cheese, but light cheese is preferable for mid-afternoon and/or pre-dinner snacks. You may parjust take in the morning refreshments. You may also appreciate additional snacks.

2 0 peanuts with their shells intact

Dipped in salad dressing or guacamole, pepper segments.

Dinner. You may consume each of the following.

Jell-O (without sugar).

salad with vinaigrette

Non-carbohydrate vegetables

Lean meat, poultry, fish, or substitute for flesh

During the first phase of the DASH diet, there are no dietary restrictions. You can consume vegetables without starch. Examples include 2 cup of leafy greens, 2 2 cup of stewed vegetables, and 6 ounces of vegetable juice. You may also consume unlimited amounts of sugar-free gelatin/Jell-O.

During Phase One, there are also some foods that can be consumed in limited quantities. Among these foods are dairy products; seeds, beans, and nuts; eggs, poultry, seafood, and lean meat; and heart-healthy fats.

During Phase One, you should avoid consuming certain substances. Included among these foods are alcoholic beverages, milk, fruit, and carbohydrate foods such as:

No foods that are batter-fried.

No starchy vegetables such as pumpkin, potatoes, or maize.

No cereals.

No foods containing flour, such as pasta or bread.

Phase II

The second phase incorporates fruits and whole cereals, as well as more dairy, lean proteins, and vegetables without starch. The objective of this phase is to allow you to maintain your weight loss momentum, albeit more progressively than in Phase One.

II. The Objective – Determining Your Dash Diet Motivation

I frequently encounter individuals who commit to regimens without a defined objective. Some refer to it as a weight loss plan, others are introduced to a diet by their nutritionist to prevent health problems, and others choose one at random from the internet. Before we embark on our voyage, I would like you to just take out a pen and paper and write down your PURPOSE for participating in Dash DIET.

Let me simplify this for you, so let's divide this into two parts.

Recommended by a dietitian or physician for X health condition(s).

I am on a mission to lose weight.

To ensure that you adhere to the plan and avoid distractions, we will now define each motive in detail based on your purpose.

The Dash Diet for Your Health

Dash Diet for YOU to Lose Weight

2 . The Dash Diet for Your Health

Originally Dash Diet was developed to control and prevent a variety of diseases. People who have a family history of certain maladies or who are on the verge of developing cardiovascular, diabetic, or cholesterol issues are recommended the Dash Diet by nutritionists. If you fall into the category of controlling or preventing health problems, you must adhere to the plan until your body's system levels stabilize.

Now, you may be wondering how long after stabilization you must adhere to the nutrition plan. The solution lies with your physician and nutritionist. Okay, you may have rolled your eyes and blasted me off a million times in your head for saying this, but believe me, it is the combined analysis of your doctor and nutritionist that will help you achieve a healthy physical state.

If you are still wondering what this book contains for you and why you should read it, the answer is that it is a COMPLETE HANDBOOK with precise information and guidance that will not allow you to deviate from your path to leading a healthy lifestyle.

The Dash Diet for Weight Loss YOU

As much as I dislike the prevalent trends of the present, I adore the fact that people are taking steps to improve their lifestyle. Unfortunately, there are too many obstacles surrounding weight loss, and I will address THREE of the FREQUENTLY ASKED QUESTIONS (FAQs) below.

Will I acquire weight if I discontinue a particular diet?

Certainly! In addition, there are no second thoughts. Diets have been criticized for their aftereffects, which include weight gain. However, you may need to realize that diets are intended to return you to a healthful state. It is an ongoing procedure that can be progressed or modified based on your physique or weight goals.

Let us demonstrate a live example RIGHT THIS MOMENT – Just take someone you admire in terms of fitness; this could be an actor, bodybuilder, fitness model, or someone you know. Examine their photographs over the years; do you notice a difference? Yes! Age plays a role, but the way you want to appear – the desired body type and weight – is what causes a transformation.

So, absolutely! Keeping note of your nutrition plan allows you to maintain a healthy weight.

Chapter 2: Instructions On Making Smoothies

Smoothies have been described as delectable, nutritious, natural, healthy, colorful, and virtually every other superlative imaginable. Smoothie consumers would readily attest to the validity of these statements. They are one of the most versatile components of a healthy diet because they can be consumed at any time of the day or night.

Smoothies are one of the simplest meals to prepare because they are essentially beverages made from a foundation mixture of fruit and vegetables that are blended to the desired consistency. Nothing could be fundamentally simpler.

However, there are a few additional guidelines that, when followed, will result in even more delicious and nutritious beverages.

It may seem obvious, but the most essential factor in creating a delicious smoothie is a high-quality blender. Your preferred blender should be a sturdy, high-quality equipment. You must ensure that the blades have a high rpm count, as this is necessary to ensure that they are capable of effectively breaking down the cellular walls of your selected vegetables, which is crucial for the release of nutrients. As a result of the likelihood that smoothies will really become a regular part of your new diet, a blender will really become one of the most essential kitchen appliances. Therefore, it is worthwhile to invest a bit more to ensure the quality and durability of your blender. It should not be viewed as a financial expense, but as an investment in your future health and well-being.

Selecting the Proper Blender.

Having established the importance of a high-quality blender, the issue now is how to select one. On the market, there are numerous varieties that all claim to be the finest at what they do. However, they all perform the same function, so how do you choose between them?

When selecting a blender, there are eight factors to consider:

2 : Power

To obtain the best results, you will need a blender with a motor that has at least 10 00 watts of power. Just keep in mind that you intend to blend vegetables with stiff skins and occasionally ice. Having a slower, less potent motor will easy make this task more difficult and produce inferior results.

2:Price

Primarily, blenders will be available in three price ranges: $6 0 or less, $80 to $2 20, and $8 00 or more for premium brands such as Vitamix and Blandtec. While it is evident that a significant portion of your decision will be based on the size of your wallet, it is still important to consider deceptive economy.

At first inspection, it may seem appealing to purchase a cheap blender, but the results may be inconsistent, resulting in smoothies with an undesirable flavor and texture. The less expensive versions are also less likely to withstand the rigors of daily use and are more likely to require frequent replacement. In essence, this means that purchasing multiple variants of the same inexpensive blender may cost you more than purchasing a single expensive blender.

I acknowledge that my opinion is subjective, but I would always recommend purchasing a mid- to high-tier product. This is the only method to ensure a high-quality smoothie with minimal effort.

6 : Pitcher/Jar.

Although it may seem unimportant, the pitcher or jar that arrives with the blender is crucial. Capacity is the most obvious cause for this. Obviously, if you have a family of two adults and two children and plan to easy make smoothies for everyone, you will need a pitcher or container with sufficient capacity to accommodate the required volume.

Pitchers and jars are made from either glass or plastic, and both materials have benefits and drawbacks that should be considered. Plastic canisters are typically lighter and more durable, but they can be difficult to clean. They have a propensity to develop scratches over time, which can serve as breeding grounds for pathogens. In contrast, glass jars tend to be heavier and more fragile, but glass is significantly simpler to clean than plastic and does not scratch as easily.

I would recommend a pitcher made from BPA-free polycarbonate whenever feasible. This combines the finest qualities of both types, as it is both shatterproof and simple to clean.

8 : Style

There is an apparent aesthetic component to this consideration, but there is also a practical component. For those with an entirely color- and style-coordinated kitchen, it is essential to have a blender that is visually appealing and complements your chosen style. When contemplating this factor, it is important to consider where you plan to store your new blender. There is no reason to purchase a blender that is too tall to suit comfortably or conveniently in your kitchen.

10 :Efficiency of Operation.

It is essential that the blender you choose can perform the desired tasks effortlessly and effectively. Smoothies are intended to be a quick and convenient substitute for snacks and even some primary meals. If a degree in astrophysics is required to operate the apparatus, then it defeats its primary purpose. It is also important to note that certain types of blenders have specialized functions such as Ice Crushing. Although these features are not essential, they surely easy make life easier, and it may be worthwhile to consider the additional cost involved.

6. Cleanup

Cleanliness is a crucial aspect of creating smoothies, and the ease with which one can effectively clean the blender is a crucial factor. It is almost certain that liquid spillage will occur during the preparation of smoothies. In these situations, it is essential to have an easy-to-clean blender. A modern blender with digital, touch-pad displays is preferable to one with push-button controls. The digital displays are much simpler to clean than their push-button counterparts, thereby simplifying the cleansing process.

Additionally, blenders with a removable blade are typically much simpler to clean than those with a fixed blade.

7:Stability

It is essential to remember that combining is a mechanical process that generates significant vibration. Whatever blender you employ must be reliable throughout this procedure. Therefore, it is essential that any blender acquired has a wide, weighty base. This will aid in preventing any residual movement or tilting during the process of blending.

8. Guarantee and Dependability

Whatever blender you decide to purchase, you will use it frequently and, ideally, for a very long time. However, nothing lasts eternally. Eventually, your blender will break down. A cheap blender will likely need to be thrown away at this stage. In the case of more expensive blenders, however, it is preferable to repair rather than replace. At the time of purchase, it is prudent to investigate the servicing and repair provisions of the manufacturer's warranty. It may be possible to purchase additional coverage at the time of purchase if necessary, and in the case of more expensive products, this may be the preferable option.

Chapter 3: A Brief Overview Of The Dash Diet

Dietary Approaches to Stop Hypertension is what "DASH" stands for in the DASH diet. The DASH diet is a lifelong approach to establishing a healthful diet that can prevent or treat hypertension (high blood pressure), as suggested by its acronym. This diet intends to reduce blood pressure by decreasing sodium injust take and increasing magnesium, calcium, and potassium intake. It also involves consuming foods with high nutritional value.

By observing the DASH diet, you can reduce your blood pressure in as little as two weeks. By sticking to the plan, you can reduce your systolic blood pressure by 8 to 2 8 points, which can help you avoid both short- and long-term health hazards.

In addition to reducing hypertension risk, the DASH diet can prevent diabetes, stroke, cardiovascular disease, cancer, and osteoporosis.

Forms of the DASH Diet

The standard DASH diet promotes regular consumption of low-fat dairy products, fruits, and vegetables and permits moderate consumption of nuts, poultry, and salmon. In addition to the standard diet, there is also a diet with less sodium, depending on your health requirements.

The standard DASH diet permits 2,6 00 milligrams of sodium per day, whereas the lower sodium DASH diet restricts sodium consumption to 2 ,10 00 mg per day. The standard DASH diet adheres to the daily sodium injust take recommendation of less than 2,6 00 mg. While the reduced sodium version serves as a maximum and is only recommended if your physician endorses it.

How to Feed

Whether you are following the standard or lower sodium version of the DASH diet, you can anticipate to consume a substantial amount of low-fat dairy products, fruits, vegetables, and whole grains. Encouraged additions include seeds and almonds, legumes, poultry, and fish a few times per week.

A standard supper on the DASH diet should be low in total fat, saturated fat, and cholesterol. To maintain a healthy diet balance, the DASH diet permits small quantities of fats, sweets, and red meat. I have listed the recommended serving sizes for a 2,000-calorie diet from each food group to help you organize your meals.

Chapter 4: The Importance Of Diet And Food

As mentioned in the preceding chapter, there are a variety of reasons why individuals will experience high blood pressure. They may have a genetic susceptibility to hypertension. It could result from their sedentary lifestyle. They could acquire it from smoking, specific medications, and other sources. There are numerous causes of elevated blood pressure, and it is frequently the result of a combination of several factors.

The foods you eat, however, are one of the most prevalent causes of hypertension. Even if you have no other risk factors for a disease, your diet can negatively affect your health, including your elevated blood pressure.

In terms of causing elevated blood pressure, the greatest problem with your diet and the foods you consume is that they contain too much salt. Convenience foods, fast foods, and freezer meals may be convenient and simple to prepare when you're occupied, but they're not the healthiest option. They contain high levels of sodium, and consuming them frequently will cause your blood pressure to rise.

Sodium by itself is not a negative substance. Your body requires sodium to maintain health, facilitate muscle function, and more. The problem arises when excessive sodium is consumed. Each day, the average American consumes 6 ,8 00 milligrams of sodium. They do not need more than 26 00 milligrams per day, and if they have high blood pressure, they could do just fine with considerably less.

All of this excess sodium comes from your diet and the foods you consume. It is unlikely that you are directly pouring salt into your mouth from the salt shaker. However, if you add a little extra salt at the dinner table or if you frequently eat out, you could easily consume this excess sodium without noticing.

There are foods that are higher in sodium than others, but the problem foods are typically those that we already know to be unhealthy. They may be simple to prepare and easy make your life easier on busy evenings, but they are slowly destroying your health.

While there are several distinct causes of high blood pressure, and some of them are difficult to control because they stem from genetics, the most common cause of high blood pressure is your diet and the foods that you enjoy eating. Understanding which foods can cause high blood pressure and how to eliminate or at least replace them can have a significant impact on your health.

43

Vegetables rich in magnesium, potassium, fiber, and other vitamins, such as verdant green vegetables, sweet potatoes, broccoli, carrots, and tomatoes, are highly recommended.

If you want to reap the full benefits of vegetables, search for recipes that can be served as a main course, such as the Bean Barley Burgers and Grilled California Veggie Sandwich. You may also serve vegetables that are fresh, chilled, or canned. However, when purchasing tinned vegetables, choose only those without added salt or those with a low sodium content.

- Cereals – The recommended number of servings of cereals per day is six to eight.

Pasta, rice, cereal, and bread are grains. One serving of grains consists of half a cup of pasta, rice, or cereal, or one slice of whole wheat bread. Whole grains are richer in nutrients and fiber than refined grains.

Focus on consuming whole grain variants, such as brown rice instead of white rice and whole wheat pasta instead of regular pasta. To maintain the low fat content of grains, avoid serving them with cheese sauces, cream, and butter.

- Dairy - The recommended number of dairy servings per day is two to three.

Although dairy is typically a significant source of fat, particularly saturated fat, the DASH diet still encourages its consumption because it is also a source of protein, vitamin D, and calcium. Cheese, yogurt, and milk are examples of dairy products, but to adhere to the DASH diet's fat consumption limit, you should choose fat-free or low-fat options. One portion of dairy can consist of any of the following: One and one-half ounces of part-skim cheese, one cup of low-fat yogurt, or one cup of skim milk.

When you're desiring a sweet snack or dessert, simply combine fruits with fat-free dairy products. Cheeses also contain sodium, so moderation is recommended. If you're lactose intolerant, you can select for lactose-free dairy products so you can still include dairy into your diet. To prevent lactose intolerance symptoms, there are over-the-counter medications containing "enzyme lactase" that effectively alleviate any undesirable signs.

- Fruits – The daily recommendation for fruit servings is four to five.

In addition to being an excellent source of magnesium, potassium, and fiber, fruits require minimal preparation to be added to a meal or eaten as a healthy snack. As with vegetables, fruits are low in cholesterol (with the exception of coconuts), so you can consume a few servings per day without feeling guilty. A single fruit serving can consist of 8 ounces of fresh juice, 1 cup of preserved, fresh, or frozen fruit, or 2 medium fruit.

How to incorporate: To meet your recommended daily fruit intake, consume one piece with each meal and one as a snack. Or you can have it as a dessert consisting of fresh blended fruits and yogurt. Additionally, if the skins are edible, just keep them on for added fiber and nutrients. Additionally, fruit peels lend interesting textures to various dishes. Choose the no-added-sugar varieties of canned fruit and beverages.

Citric acids found in fruits and beverages may interact negatively with certain medications. If you just take medications on a regular basis, consult your doctor to determine if you should limit or avoid certain fruits.

- Fish, Poultry, and Lean Meat – The recommended number of daily servings for fish, poultry, and lean meat is six.

A single serving of fish, poultry, or lean meat should not exceed 2 ounce on the DASH diet. By reducing the amount of meat, you can easy make space for more vegetables.

When preparing meat and poultry, it is necessary to remove the skin and trim the fat. Easy cook using roasting, grilling, broiling, or baking rather than lard. Choose varieties of fish that are known to be beneficial for the heart, such as tuna, herring, and salmon. Because they contain Omega-6 fatty acids, these types of fish can lower cholesterol.

- Oils and Fats - The daily recommendation for oils and fats is two to three servings.

As is common knowledge, lipids have a high caloric content and can contribute to obesity, diabetes, and heart disease. However, lipids are essential components of a healthy diet. In fact, they can enhance the immune system by facilitating the absorption of essential nutrients and vitamins. In order to maintain a healthy balance, the DASH diet permits a maximum fat injust take of 6 0% per day. 2 tablespoons of salad dressing, 2 tablespoon of mayonnaise, or 2 teaspoon of soft margarine comprise a single serving of oils and lipids.

To avoid unhealthy lipids, restrict your consumption of butter, eggs, meat, cream, whole milk, and cheese. Additionally, avoid foods that contain or are made with palm or coconut oil, solid shortening, and lard. Also containing trans-fat are processed foods such as fried foods, baked products, and crackers; avoid these as much as possible. Check the nutrition labels to determine which foods are low in saturated and trans fats if you are uncertain.

- Legumes, Seeds, and Nuts – The recommended number of servings of legumes, seeds, and nuts per week is four to five.

This category of foods is rich in protein, potassium, and magnesium. Included in this category are lentils, peas, kidney beans, sunflower seeds, and hazelnuts. In addition to vitamins and nutrients, this food group is rich in fiber and phytochemicals that protect against cardiovascular disease and certain malignancies. One serving of nuts, seeds, and legumes can consist of half a cup of cooked peas or beans, two tablespoons of seeds, or one-third of a cup of nuts.

How to implement: Because nuts are high in calories and fats, most regimens prohibit their consumption. Nonetheless, they also contain heart-healthy Omega-6 fatty acids. This form of food can be used as a topping for cereals, salads, and stir-fries. You can also obtain your servings by substituting soy products such as tempeh and tofu for meat.

- desserts - The recommended amount of desserts per week is five or less servings.

In order to maintain a balanced diet, you should still consume a couple of servings of desserts. 2 cup of lemonade, 2 2 cup of sorbet, or 2 tablespoon of jam or jelly can constitute a single serving of desserts.

If you have a sweet tooth, you can indulge in cookies, crackers, hard chocolates, jelly beans, and sorbets, but it would be beneficial to choose the low-fat or fat-free varieties over the regular ones. To reduce sugar intake, you can also use artificial sweeteners like

Splenda and Equal when preparing desserts or sweet munchies.

Chapter 5: Alcohol And Caffeine: Their Effects

Alcohol consumption can increase blood pressure. Therefore, the DASH diet emphasizes the importance of limiting alcohol consumption. Men are limited to two servings of alcohol per day, while women are limited to one. Caffeine's effect on blood pressure is still unknown, as individuals appear to have varying levels of caffeine tolerance. If consuming caffeinated beverages causes your blood pressure to rise, even temporarily, you should consult a physician for advice.

DASH Diet and Losing Weight

Despite the fact that the DASH diet is not intended for weight loss, you may still lose weight by making healthier food choices and counting calories. The standard DASH diet allows you to consume 2,000 calories per day. If you wish to lose weight, you may consume fewer calories than recommended; however, you should first consult your doctor, as a sudden reduction in caloric consumption may also cause a dangerous change in your blood pressure.

French toast with apple butter

2 teaspoon of ground cinnamon

12 slices of whole wheat bread

1 cup of unsweetened applesauce

2 cup of milk

4 fresh eggs

4 tablespoons of white sugar

Directions:

1.   Mix applesauce, sugar, cinnamon, milk, and fresh eggs until thoroughly-combined.
2.   Soak the bread, a piece at a time, until the mixture is absorbed slightly.
3.   Set a lightly greased skillet over medium heat and easy cook the soaked bread slices until both sides are golden brown.
4. Serve while still hot.

Papaya And Coconut Shake

4 tbsp. wheat germ
 2 tsp. zero-calorie sugar (optional)

2 ready papaya, cultivated, stripped,
and cut into 2 -inch
 lumps 2 cup plain low-fat yogurt
 2 cup coconut water (not coconut milk)

DIRECTIONS

1. Combine all ingredients, including sweetener (if using), in a blender.

2. Fill two tall glasses and serve.

Peach And Fruit Crêpe

 2 cup new raspberries
4 medium peaches 2 tsp. sugar

2 cup generally useful flour
1 cup vanilla yogurt
1/7 tsp. salt
2 tbsp. butter
2 cup without fat milk
6 enormous fresh eggs

Directions

1.
    Put the raspberries, peaches, and sugar in a bowl.

2. Tenderly throw to cover.

3. Put milk, eggs, and salt in a bowl. Rush until joined.

4. Progressively add flour as you whisk. Place spread in a pie plate and soften in a preheated stove at 450°F for 5 to 10 minutes.

5. Eliminate from the stove and spread softened margarine everywhere.

6. Add the player and heat for 40 to 45 minutes or until carmelized and puffed.

7. Top with yogurt and blended fruits.

Chapter 6: Benefits Of Dash Diet

Nutrition is an integral part of hypertension or high blood pressure management, both in terms of prevention and treatment. The DASH diet, also known as "Dietary Approaches to Stop Hypertension," is frequently recommended by healthcare professionals.

The DASH diet, which has been shown in multiple studies to be effective in regulating blood pressure in patients with hypertension and pre-hypertension, produces results in as little as two weeks. In addition, researchers have discovered over the past two decades that the DASH diet is beneficial for lowering cholesterol, protecting cardiac health, lowering the risk of type 2 diabetes, and lowering the risk of developing certain types of cancer. Due to the DASH diet's emphasis on fruits and vegetables, whole grains, lean proteins, and healthy lipids, all of these benefits are realized.

The DASH diet is heart-healthy.

In addition to reducing inflammation and blood pressure, the DASH diet also reduces cholesterol and triglyceride levels, all of which are cardiovascular disease risk factors. In a meta-analysis of over 480 studies, the DASH diet was found to be associated with a reduced risk of cardiovascular disease, coronary heart disease, and stroke. A meta-analysis is a large-scale study that compiles data from multiple investigations on the same topic.

The consumption of a diet rich in plant-based foods, such as vegetables, fruits, grains, legumes, and seeds, is largely responsible for the cardiovascular health benefits. To obtain the benefits of the DASH diet for your heart health, however, you do not have to eliminate all animal-based foods. The DASH diet permits moderate quantities of poultry, fish, eggs, lean meat, and dairy products in addition to plant-based foods. Discover the specific dietary recommendations provided here.

The Dietary Approach to Stop Hypertension (DASH) program also recommends at least thirty minutes of physical activity on the majority of days. This provides an additional layer of cardiac protection.

DASH vs. malignancy

Other researchers were interested in determining whether or not individuals who followed the DASH diet to treat hypertension would experience any additional benefits. It appears there are many of them! A meta-analysis of the protective effect of the DASH diet against various types of cancer, including colorectal, breast, hepatic, endometrial, and lung cancer, was conducted using a total of 12 7 separate studies. There was a correlation between strict adherence to the DASH diet and a reduced mortality rate from all of these cancer types. Diabetes type 2 versus DASH

The Dietary Approaches to Stop Hypertension in its Advanced Stages (DASH) is also one of the most recommended dietary patterns to help avoid type 2 diabetes. Consumption of low-fat dairy, yogurt, olive oil, and whole grains, as well as adequate intakes of fiber and magnesium, are credited by the study's authors. They also highlight the preventive effect of flavonoid antioxidants, which can be obtained by consuming a diet rich in fruits and vegetables.

The DASH diet also places restrictions on foods that are high in refined sugars and refined flours, both of which contribute to an increase in blood sugar levels due to their high glycemic index. A significant increase in the risk of developing type 2 diabetes is associated with consuming large amounts of refined flour, sugary foods, and red or processed meat; however, the DASH diet is low in all of these foods, providing a preventive benefit.

The DASH diet is a great option not just for lowering or maintaining blood pressure, but also for anyone seeking a healthy, varied, and delicious diet.

Chapter 7: Lean Meat, Poultry, Fish, And Various Substitutes

These are important contributors of protein and magnesium to the DASH diet and dietary staples for many. Vegans and vegetarians can confidently replace the animal-based protein sources outlined here with legume-based proteins such as tofu, lentils, and chickpeas, among others. Beef tenderloin, sirloin, and eye of round contain less fat than other commonly available cuts. Additionally, avoiding purchasing cuts with visible fat and trimming fat prior to easily cooking are beneficial. We recommend eating multiple servings of fish each week.

12 ounces of cooked meat, poultry, or fish, 12 eggs, and 36 ounces of tofu constitute one serving.

NUTS, SEEDS, AND LEGUMES

This group of foods is distinctive due to the fact that they are among the relatively small group of plant-based foods that contain both iron and protein, two essential nutrients that animal proteins provide. In contrast to most types of meat, however, these options are rich in fiber and heart-healthy monounsaturated fat while containing significantly less saturated fat.

Size of a serving: 13 cup raw or unsalted nuts or seeds, 2 teaspoons nut butter, and 12 cups cooked legumes (preferably cooked from raw, as canned legumes are higher in sodium).

HEALTHY FATS AND OILS

This category comprises the types of foods we may use to garnish or prepare food. When people think of healthful fats, they frequently consider olive oil and other vegetable oils, which are excellent options and far superior to lard and butter. However, it is important to be mindful of how much of these items we consume because, in addition to being high in calories, many of the nutritional benefits of oils can be found in greater quantities in foods such as nuts and seeds, which also contain fiber and just keep us feeling satiated. We recommend creating your own salad vinaigrette with oil and vinegar. If purchasing from a store, choose the refrigerated versions and be sure to read the labels and select the version with the least amount of sodium. We also provide healthier salad dressing recipes in our recipe section.

12 teaspoons of oil, 2 tablespoons of light salad dressing, and 12 tablespoons of standard salad dressing easy make up one serving.

MORE ON OILS The majority of our fat injust take from oils should consist of unsaturated lipids, while some saturated fats are acceptable. Avoiding trans fats, also known as hydrogenated oils, is advised. Depending on the type of fatty acids in oils and how they were processed, each has a unique smoke point or burn point, requiring the use of distinct oils for various applications.

• Use neutral unsaturated oils, such as canola or avocado oil, when easily cooking with high heat, such as roasting, stir-frying, or barbecuing. Canola is reasonably priced and contains omega-36 fatty acids. Avocado is an excellent alternative, as it is composed primarily of monounsaturated fatty acids and has the highest combustion point of all oils, but it is more expensive. Both are superb easily cooking oils; it depends on personal preference and budget. These oils are suitable for the majority of recipes in this book. I've included "canola oil" in the recipes because it's the least costly option, but feel free to use your preferred oil. Choose organic canola oil if you wish to avoid genetically modified organisms (GMOs), as any product labeled organic must also be free of GMOs by law.

• Use extra-virgin olive oil, which is high in monounsaturated fats, when easily cooking with moderate heat, such as a quick sauté, or when preparing the majority of salad dressings. It has a low smoke point, so avoid roasting, stir-frying, and grilling at high temperatures.

When an oil begins to ignite, its chemical composition changes, rendering it potentially unhealthy. Other olive oils, such as extra light, are refined differently and have a higher smoke point. If you prefer the flavor of olive oil, you can also use these oils for high-heat cookery. I appreciate using olive oil in Mediterranean-style dishes, as the flavor complements the cuisine well. Olive oil is indicated where it is most applicable in this book.

There are many other nutritious oils available on the market besides the ones I've listed above. To just keep things basic and affordable, we've shared with you a handful of oils that we use frequently due to their nutritional qualities and culinary applications.

We should also discuss coconut oil given its recent popularity. Given that it is both a saturated fat and a plant, and that studies on it are conflicting, we generally recommend consuming it occasionally, such as when creating granola bar recipes or baking.

SWEETS

The fact that you can eat dessert is the final proof that the DASH diet is unlike any other diet you've likely attempted. Yes, you may consume treats, and you may do so more than once per week. Unfortunately, the restrictive nature of many diets makes them difficult to maintain for many individuals. The DASH diet is a long-term, sustainable eating regimen that encourages both food and life enjoyment. Don't fret, ice cream can still be consumed in moderation.

12 ounces of ice cream or frozen yogurt; 12 tablespoons of nectar, honey, or sugar; 12 ounces of juice or other sugar-sweetened beverage per serving.easily cooking easy cook just keep just take easily cooking easily cooking easily cooking easily cooking easily cooking just keep

Sodium, commonly referred to as the salt found in or added to food, is frequently ingested in excess and is one of the primary causes of high blood pressure. Detailed strategies for adhering to the daily sodium injust take limit of 2,3600 milligrams will be presented in the following section.

Goal: Beginning with less than 2,360,000 milligrams per day (12 teaspoon), gradually increase to no more than 12,510,00 milligrams per day (34 teaspoon).

LOWER-SODIUM LIVING

In some individuals, protracted excessive sodium injust take contributes to high blood pressure by causing chronic fluid retention, which ultimately strains the blood vessels. However, reducing the amount of salt in your diet might not be as simple as putting the shaker away. In reality, the majority of individuals will require a multifaceted strategy to significantly reduce their daily intake. Let's examine in greater detail the three areas where this can be accomplished most effectively:

When shopping for food: Your mission to reduce the quantity of sodium in your diet begins at the supermarket. Any food product sold in a package or a bottle, from crackers to pasta sauces, has the potential to have a very high sodium content. Utilizing the labels on these products to compare the sodium content of foods within the same category is your best defense. Selecting the item with the lowest sodium content is an excellent starting point.

At house: Did you know that a teaspoon of salt contains your daily sodium limit (2,360 milligrams) for the DASH diet? Those who don't add salt to their cuisine need not worry, but if you are a frequent user, you should be concerned. It may be time to rely on herbs, spices, or sodium-free mixtures of the two. When combined with acidic flavors, such as those provided by lemon juice or vinegar, you won't miss a thing in terms of flavor and will ultimately require less sodium-laden condiments from the store. The greatest part is that part 2 of this book contains 12,000 delectable lower-sodium recipes. Dining out As compared to home-cooked meals, the sodium content of any given restaurant entrée is likely to be substantially higher. This is problematic for those with hypertension, and it is particularly problematic for sauce-heavy pasta dishes. French fries and various soups may be examples of additional severely salted restaurant fare. Consequently, establishing weekly objectives for the number of meals you eat out is a crucial component of your future lifestyle.

just take just take easy make just take

Chapter 8: Kick-Start Your Dash Diet Weight-Loss Program

Up until now, I've walked you through the fundamentals of the DASH diet while also explaining why it tends to be your key to intelligent dietary success. However, learning does not end here. As we progress through this book, more of your questions regarding modified nutrition, calories, exercise, and meal preparation will be addressed.

You will not only learn about the DASH diet, but also how to integrate its principles into your daily life to provide a long-term solution to your health issues. I am aware that weight loss is at the forefront of your mind, so we will continue this journey by discussing in greater detail why weight loss can be so difficult and how you can use the inclusivity of the DASH diet to overcome many of the difficulties you may have encountered in the past with restrictive diets.

From there, I will lead you into a discussion of the multitude of other significant aspects of your all-encompassing approach to welness, including procedures for further developed rest, exercise, and stress management, all of which will assist you in maximizing the benefits of the DASH diet.

You will, despite everything, learn how to advance your eating habits through the use of pranks and tasty recipes. The 28-day plan that is just around the corner will allow you to effortlessly incorporate the DASH diet standards into your daily life and outline the path to long-term success.

Everything begins now.

2 Tackling Weight Loss

The greatest aspect of the DASH diet is that it can provide you with a healthy, balanced path to weight loss. However, weight reduction is difficult, and maintaining weight loss is even more difficult.

They may rely on unrealistic dietary examples, which contributes to the fact that many individuals may struggle to get fit or maintain their weight loss. Fortunately, one of the most notable characteristics of the DASH diet is that it is a sustainable, unrestrictive, and relatively easy-to-follow strategy for weight loss. In this section, you'll learn more about the science behind weight loss, as well as commonsense strategies for addressing your assumptions and increasing your chances of success.

just take easy make just keep

Couscous Salad With Salmon

- 8 ounces of cooked salmon

- 1/2 cup dried apricots, sliced

- 1 ounce of crumbled goat cheese, about 4 tablespoons

- 1/2 cup of sliced cremini mushrooms

- 1 cup diced eggplant

- 6 servings of baby spinach

- Divide the 4 tablespoons of white wine vinaigrette (see Tip)

- 1/2 cup cooked Israeli couscous, whole-wheat couscous is best.

1. Spray easily cooking spray on a small skillet and heat it over medium-high heat.
2. Add the mushrooms and eggplant and stir-fry for 10 to 15 minutes, until they are lightly browned and the juices have come out.
3. Just take it off the heat and set it aside.
4. Mix 2 Tbsp. plus 2 tsp. vinaigrette and put it on a 9-inch plate.
5. Mix the couscous with the other 4 tsp. Put the vinaigrette on top cf the spinach.]
6. Salmon goes on top.
7. Goat cheese, dried apricots, and the cooked vegetables go on top.

easy make just keep

Cauliflower Hash

4 cups cauliflower, riced or chopped in
food processor
Pepper to Taste
4 tbsp butter

2 onion diced
2 red pepper diced
2 cup shredded corned beef
4 cups cooked sweet potato, diced

Directions:

Melt the butter over medium heat and easy cook the onion in it until it is translucent. Stir in the capsicum and cauliflower. Add the beef after 5 to 10 minutes of easily cooking the vegetables. Stir the mixture thoroughly before adding sweet potatoes. With a spatula, press the potato mixture firmly into the pan so that the potatoes hold everything together. Allow the underside of the patty to brown and really become crisp before flipping. Once the other side is crisp, remove the hash and serve.

easy cook

Sweet Potato Porridge

1 cup fresh blueberries
2 tbsp honey
2 tsp cinnamon

2 sweet potato, peeled and diced
2 cup steel cut oats
2 tbsp chia seeds
8 strawberries hulled and quartered

Directions:

1. In a medium saucepan cover the potatoes with water and then bring them to a boil over medium-high heat.
2. Easy cook the potatoes for 10 minutes and then drain. Easy cook the oatmeal according to package directions and then stir in the honey and cinnamon.
3. Add the chia seed and most of the sweet potato.
4. Warm the oatmeal through on low-medium heat and then divide it into two bowls.
5. Top with fruit and remaining potato.

Chapter 9: Additional Potential Health Benefits

Reduce cancer risk: A recent study found that those who followed the DASH diet had a lower risk of certain cancers, including soloretal and breast cancer. Reduced metabolic syndrome risk: Some studies indicate that the DASH diet reduces the risk of metabolic syndrome by 812%. The diet has been associated with a decreased incidence of type 2 diabetes. Some studies demonstrate that it can also promote neuronal regeneration. Reduce the risk of heart disease: In a recent study on women, following a DASH-like diet was associated with a 20% reduction in the risk of heart disease and a 29% reduction in the risk of stroke. Many of these health benefits can be attributed to the diet's high fruit and vegetable content. In general, eating more fruits and vegetables san helr reduse risk of disease.

DASH LOWERS BLOOD RRESSURE — unusual if you have elevated levels — and you are underweight. It should reduce your risk of diabetes, heart disease, metabolic disorder, and certain cancers.

DOES IT WORK FOR ALL PEOPLE?

While studies on the DASH diet determined that those with the lowest salt intake experienced the greatest reductions in blood pressure, the benefits of sodium restriction on health and longevity are unclear. For individuals with high blood pressure, reducing salt intake has a significant impact on blood pressure. However, in individuals with normal blood pressure, reducing salt intake has much smaller effects.The theory that certain receptors are alt entve — meaning that alt exerts a greater influence on their blood rreure — could possibly explain this. If your sodium intake is high, reducing it can have significant health benefits. However, comprehensive sodium restriction, as recommended by the DASH diet, may only be beneficial for individuals who are sodium sensitive or have high blood pressure.

TOO MUCH SALT RESTRICTION IS NOT GOOD FOR YOU

Eating too little salt has been linked to health issues, such as an increased risk of cardiac disease, high blood pressure, and fluid retention. The low-sodium version of the DASH diet suggests that individuals consume no more than 36/48 teaspoon (12,510 mg) of sodium per day. However, it is unclear whether there are any benefits to reducing salt intake to extremely low levels, even in individuals with high blood pressure. A recent study found no link between salt intake and the risk of dying from heart disease, despite the fact that reducing salt intake led to a moderate reduction in blood pressure.

However, because most people consume too much salt, reducing your salt intake from extremely high amounts of 2–2.510 tearoon (12 0–12 2 gram) per day to 12–12.2510 tearoon (510–6 gram) per day may be beneficial. The goal can be easily attained by reducing the amount of highly processed foods in your diet and eating primarily whole foods.

Chapter 10: What Benefits Does The Dash Diet Offer?

If you want to attempt the DASH diet, there are no disadvantages because it consists of eating the healthiest foods and reducing your intake of unhealthy foods. In addition to aiding in weight loss, it helps maintain "heart health, blood pressure, and cholesterol levels"

Almost everyone would benefit from consuming less sodium and more nutritious foods. Due to the importance of vegetables in the DASH diet, I like to prepare roasted lemon pepper asparagus to accompany a lean protein such as tofu. Additionally, spaghetti squash is a suitable substitute for pasta.

Due to its emphasis on fresh, nutritious foods, the DASH diet is not only beneficial for lowering blood pressure, but also for weight loss, gaining energy, and feeling better in general. Additionally, it can help reduce lipids and manage or prevent diabetes.

Benefit from the advantages of a nutritious diet. The DASH diet consists of a variety of nutritious and tasty dishes. Even if you don't have hypertension, DASH can help you maintain a healthy diet and lifestyle.

By adhering to the DASH recommendations, you will also increase your intake of calcium, magnesium, and fiber, all of which are essential for good health.

The most apparent advantage of the DASH diet is its ability to significantly reduce hypertension. It has been found to reduce blood pressure by eight to twelve and forty-eight points. Additionally, it was discovered that this diet benefits the health of individuals with type 2 diabetes and chronic heart disease.

In addition, since the nutritional plans have been modified, those who adhere to this diet may experience weight loss. Increased protein consumption and the substitution of refined carbohydrates with whole grains have been linked to weight loss with preservation of muscle mass.

This nutrition plan has been ranked as the greatest diet ever due to the numerous health benefits experienced by those who have followed it. Due to the vast array of health and well-being benefits that the Dash Diet provides, it consistently stands apart from other diets.

Why the Dash Diet is beneficial to your health:

You reduce your blood pressure by 12 points

Clearly, this is the primary benefit of the DASH diet, as it is designed specifically to attain this objective. This diet is an excellent choice for those who are presently taking blood pressure medication or who wish to better manage the symptoms of prehypertension.

Second, you will consume healthier foods

People who have never spent a significant amount of time in the kitchen will need to acclimate to this. But with all the fresh produce you'll be consuming and the decrease in processed foods, you'll be able to experience much tastier, more nutritious meals.

Spend some time experimenting with new fruits and vegetables, as well as salt-free condiments, in order to prepare nutritious meals that your family will appreciate. Instead of a quick sandwich or fast-food burger, a little planning and concentration on the DASH diet will allow you to experience significantly more nutritious foods.

You possess healthier cholesterol levels.

Your cholesterol levels will improve as a result of the fiber you obtain from fruits and vegetables, whole grains, nuts, and legumes, as well as the lean meat and fish you consume and the limited amount of sweets and refined carbohydrates you consume. This enhancement persists with a diet higher in fat, which also increases "good" cholesterol.

You will adore Dash and stay with him.

Because this diet consists of readily available, delectable foods, it is very simple for the majority of individuals to adhere to. Now that you have decided to follow the DASH diet, you can enjoy permanent lifestyle modifications that are beneficial to your overall health and well-being.

The DASH diet is simple to adhere to even when dining out. Simply observe which foods are sabotaging your efforts. There are numerous methods in which the DASH diet can lead to success. This is an enormous benefit for anyone seeking to enhance their health.

You will experience optimal weight maintenance

Whether or not you wish to lose weight, the DASH diet is an excellent option for achieving your weight-loss objective. A modified variant of the DASH diet can help you achieve your weight loss objectives. Then, increase your caloric intake to maintain your new weight.

The DASH diet is strong in protein without excessive carbohydrate consumption. You enjoy building muscle and revving up your metabolism without ever feeling weighty. This is not a temporary diet, but a new, healthful lifestyle.

You reduce the possibility of developing osteoporosis.

The majority of nutritional strategies used to prevent and treat osteoporosis involve increasing your intake of vitamin D and calcium, both of which are abundant in many DASH diet ingredients. Additionally, research has demonstrated that sodium reduction is an effective strategy. Therefore, the DASH diet has additional benefits for bone health.

Your kidneys will be more healthy

Due to the foods' potassium, magnesium, fiber, and calcium content, the Dash Diet reduces the risk of developing kidney disease and kidney stones. People who are at risk of developing kidney disease are also advised to follow a diet that emphasizes reduced sodium consumption.

However, patients diagnosed with chronic kidney disease or on dialysis should not follow this diet without the guidance of a healthcare professional, as these patients may have special restrictions.

You are better protected against certain cancer varieties.

The researchers examined the relationship between the DASH diet and various types of cancer and discovered a positive association between reducing sodium intake and monitoring fat consumption and a decreased risk of cancer. Additionally, the diet is limited in red meat, which has been linked to colon, rectum, esophagus, stomach, lungs, prostate, and kidney cancers.

Focusing on fresh produce and low-fat dairy products can prevent a number of malignancies and reduce the risk of colon cancer, respectively.

9th: Diabetes is preventable

It has been demonstrated that the DASH diet is an effective method for preventing diabetes. It has been shown to be associated with cardiovascular health hazards and high blood pressure. The DASH diet helps to control sodium intake, increase fiber and potassium consumption, and maintain a healthy weight. Thus, Dash aids those predisposed to diabetes in preventing or delaying its onset.

According to a number of studies, this effect is amplified when the DASH diet is incorporated into an overall healthy lifestyle that includes diet, exercise, and weight management.

You will no longer experience hunger.

Due to its high fiber and protein content, the DASH diet will never induce appetites for unhealthy foods. You will feel satisfied throughout the day and anticipate your next nutritious, filling meal. Nevertheless, it is prudent to prepare in advance. In order to stay on track by consuming DASH-approved snacks, you should ultimately really become famished.

Low-fat diets and carbohydrate restriction can cause hunger. However, since you are pleased with the DASH diet and achieving success with it, it will be much simpler to maintain in the long term.

12 12th will easy make you feel and look youthful.

Numerous adherents of this diet assert that the DASH eating plan will assist them in delaying the onset of certain effects of aging. These individuals continually appear and feel youthful as time passes.

By consuming more fresh fruits and vegetables that are rich in beneficial antioxidants, you will lose weight and feel healthier while rejuvenating your skin and hair, bones, joints, and muscles.

You will experience improved mental health

Improving your mood and reducing the symptoms of disorders such as depression or anxiety can be attributed to the lifestyle effects of the DASH diet, which include exercise, moderate alcohol consumption, and cigarette avoidance.

However, the nutrient-dense foods recommended in this diet promote mental health and well-being by balancing the chemicals and hormones in the brain and body.

12 36th: You have a more robust cerebral function.

Researchers have discovered that the DASH diet can just keep your brain healthy and even prevent memory loss as you age, thereby reducing the rate of mental decline. Additionally, the DASH-recommended low-fat, high-fiber diet plan reduces blood pressure. This is a documented risk factor for degenerative diseases like Alzheimer's and dementia.

According to research, the greatest foods for preventing mental decline are vegetables, whole grains, low-fat dairy products, legumes, and nuts - the main components of the DASH diet.

You reduce the likelihood of developing cardiac disease.

Due to the unique ability of the DASH diet to lower and control blood pressure, adhering to this diet can significantly increase your body's resistance to cardiac disease. A 2012 study discovered that the DASH diet can "significantly" reduce a person's risk of developing coronary artery disease, which researchers deem to be of great public health benefit given the enormous and persistent burden of coronary artery disease.

The lowered blood pressure allows the heart to function more effectively and efficiently, but it can also be beneficial for those who do not have high blood pressure but wish to prevent the development of heart disease.

12 510. You have an improved and healthier lifestyle.

The DASH diet is not only about healthy eating, but also about taking manageable measures to control your own health and wellness. By incorporating diet, exercise, and healthy living into your lifestyle, you will obtain a number of additional valuable benefits in addition to the health advantages of DASH dining.

Begin gradually and practice consuming the DASH-recommended foods. Really become accustomed to dishes without as much added salt. Exercise multiple times per week. Limit your intake of alcoholic beverages and desserts. Soon, following the DASH diet will really become second nature, and maintaining a healthy lifestyle will be effortless.

just keep easy make easy make just keep easy make just keep easy make

- French toast with apple butter 4 tablespoons white sugar

- 2 /8 cup unsweetened applesauce

- 12 slices whole wheat bread 4 fresh eggs

- 1 cup milk

- 2 teaspoon ground cinnamon

-

1. Mix eggs, milk, cinnamon, sugar and applesauce in a bowl.

2. Soak bread until mixture is absorbed.

3. Easy cook on lightly greased skillet over medium heat until golden brown on both sides.

4. Serve hot.

Baked Oatmeal

Ingredients

- 4 fresh eggs
- 4 tsp vanilla
- 1/2 cup brown sugar
- 4 cups Quick Quaker Oats
- 1/2 cup granulated sugar
- 1 tsp salt
- 1-2 cups fat-free milk

1. Preheat oven to 350 F.

2. Spray a baking dish with easily cooking spray.

3. Mix oats, granulated sugar and salt in a bowl.

4. Mix milk, fresh eggs and vanilla in a different bowl.

5. Add to oat mixture and mix well.

6. Pour into baking dish.

7. Bake for 70 to 80 minutes.

8. Sprinkle brown sugar evenly over top of oatmeal before serving.

Energy Sunrise Muffins

Ingredients:

4 teaspoons vanilla extract 4 cups shredded carrots
 2 large apple, peeled and grated
 2 cup golden raisins
 2 cup chopped pecans
 2 cup unsweetened coconut flakes

Nonstick easily cooking spray 4 cups whole wheat flour 4 teaspoons baking soda
 4 teaspoons ground cinnamon 2 teaspoon ground ginger 1 teaspoon salt
6 large eggs
 2 cup packed brown sugar
 ½ cup unsweetened applesauce
 1 cup honey
 1 cup vegetable or canola oil 2

teaspoon grated orange zest Juice of 2 medium orange

Directions:

1. If you can fit two 1-5-cup biscuit tins one next to the other in your broiler, then, at that point, leave the rack in the center.
2. In any case, position racks in the upper and lower the stove and preheat the broiler to 350°F.
3. Coat 30 cups of the biscuit tins with easily cooking shower or line with paper   li
In a huge bowl, consolidate the flour, baking pop, cinnamon, ginger, and Set aside.

4. In a medium bowl, whisk together the eggs, earthy colored sugar, fruit

purée, h oil, orange zing, squeezed orange, and vanilla until joined.
5. Add the carrot apple and whisk once more.
Blend the dry and wet fixings in with a spatula.
6. Overlap in the raise walnuts and coconut.
7. Blend everything indeed, just until well   combined.

8. Spoon the hitter into the biscuit cups, filling   them   to   the   top.

9. Bake for 45 to 50   minutes, or until a wooden toothpick embedded into the center of the middle biscuit confesses all.
10.   Just cool for 10 to 15   minutes in the tins, moves to a wire rack to just cool for 5-10   extra minutes.
11.   Just cool totally prior to putting away in containers.

12.   Storage: Cover extra biscuits, and store at room temperature for 4 days or in the cooler for multi week.
13.   May freeze as long as multi month and defrost in the fridge short-term before   serving.

14.   Sans   gluten   choice: Use universally handy sans gluten flour.

Uncomplicated Cheese And Broccoli Omelets

Ingredients:

2 teaspoon freshly ground black pepper
16 tablespoons shredded reduced-fat
Monterey Jack cheese, divided

6 tablespoons extra-virgin olive oil,
divided 4 cups chopped broccoli
16 large eggs
1 cup 2 % milk

Directions:

1. In   a   nonstick   skillet,   heat   2
   tablespoon of oil over medium-high
   hotness.

119

2. Broccoli and sauté, sometimes mixing, for 10 to 15   minutes, or until the broccoli really really become a striking shade of green.
3. Scratch into a bowl.
4. In a little bowl, beat together the eggs,   milk,   and   pepper.

5. Wipe out the skillet and hotness 2 tablespoon of oil.
6. Add onefourth of the blend and slant the skillet to guarantee an even layer.
7. Easy cook for 1-5 minutes a then add 4   tablespoons   of   cheddar   and onefourth of the broccoli.
8. Utilize a spatula to overlap into an omelet.
   Repeat stage 5-10 with the excess 1-5 tablespoons of oil, remaining fresh egg blend, 12 tablespoons of cheddar, and remaining broccoli to easy make an absolute omelet. Partition into 8 stockpiling containers. Storage: Store in the cooler for as long as 10 days.

9. To warm, microwave for 60 seconds to 2 moment, prepare at 350 °F for as long as 20 minutes, or hotness in a skillet with a smidgen of olive oil until warm.

Italian Sausage Zucchini Boats

Vegetable   oil
2   cup   Panko   breadcrumbs
4   tablespoons   oregano,   minced
4   tablespoons   basil,   minced
4 medium, cored, sliced tomatoes

12 medium zucchini

1/2   cup Parmesan grated Cheese
1-2   cup   minced   parsley
1-2   teaspoon ground black pepper
1/2   cup   part-skim   shredded
mozzarella   cheese
Italian sausage 2 lb, casing removed

1. Preheat oven to 350 degrees F. Cut zucchini in half along the length.
2. Then scoop out 1/2 of the pulp to easy   make   a   boat.

3. Place the zucchini boats in a microwave safe oven, one per batch

depending on the capacity of the microwave.

4. Turn on the microwave to medium heat and easy cook covered for 5-10 minutes.

5. Heat vegetable oil in a skillet to easy cook the zucchini pulp and sausage for 15 to 20 minutes.

6. Once the sausage is cooked, break it upto   bite-sized.

7.

8. Toss   in   tomatoes,   Panko breadcrumbs or Parmesan cheese.

9. Add   pepper   and   other   herbs.

10.   Place the filling on the zucchini boats.

11.   Place the zucchini boats on a baking sheet and bake in the microwave   oven.

12.   20   minutes.

Sprinkle mozzarella cheese on the oven and bake covered for 15 to 20 minutes, until   it   melts.
Just take the baking sheet out of the oven and garnish with chopped parsley.

Turkey Barbecue Burger

2 thinly sliced tomato
 2 slice provolone cheese
 2 Red onion sliced thinly
 4 tablespoons oat bran
 6 Two tablespoons barbecue sauce with smokey flavor 8 Split whole wheat hamburger buns

1/2   cup chopped basil
 1/2   teaspoon garlic salt
1/7 teaspoon ground pepper

Ground turkey 2 lb lean
2 clove minced garlic

Preparation

1. In a bowl, combine barbecue sauce, oat Bran, garlic, salt, pepper, and basil.

2. Easy make burger patties 1 inch thick by adding ground turkey. Lightly grease a grill pan with vegetable oil.

Grill Hamburger Buns Until Golden Brown.
Place The Turkey Patties With Your Favorite   Toppings.
Serve On A Platter. The Ultimate Green Salad

- **Ingredients** 1 cup roughly chopped roasted red peppers
- 6 tbsp red wine vinegar
- 4 tbsp olive oil
- 2 tsp grainy mustard
- 2 tsp maple syrup
- Kosher salt and freshly ground pepper, to taste

- 16 cups fresh kale, tough ribbing removed, chopped

- 2 cup cooked quinoa

- 2 cup cooked green lentils 2 cup frozen, shelled edamame, defrosted

Directions

1. Place kale, quinoa, lentils, edamame, and roasted red peppers in a large bowl.

2. In a small bowl, whisk together vinegar, olive oil, mustard, maple syrup, salt, and pepper.
3. Pour over salad and toss to evenly coat.

Pumpkin Pancakes

Ingredients:

- 2 small egg
- 2 Tbsp coconut sugar or Stevia
- 1 Tbsp baking powder
- 1 tsp salt
- 1 tsp pumpkin pie spice
- 2 cup almond or whole wheat flour
- 1/2 cup nonfat milk
- 2 Tbsp flax seed or canola oil
- 1/2 cup pureed pumpkin, fresh or canned

How to Prepare:

1. Beat the fresh egg in a bowl until frothy, then whisk in the milk and oil.

2. Slowly mix in the baking powder, salt, flour, sugar or Stevia, and spice.

3. Do not over-mix.

4. Place a nonstick skillet over medium flame and use a ladle to pour some of the batter onto it.

5. Easy cook for 1-5 minute per side or until firm, then transfer to a plate.

6. Repeat until you have used up all the batter. Serve warm.

French Toast That Satisfies

Ingredients:

- 2 small egg
- 1/2 cup nonfat milk
- 1/2 tsp pure vanilla extract
- Apple pie spice
- 8 slices of whole wheat French bread, 2 inch thick each
- 1/2 cup nonfat cream cheese
- 2 Tbsp unsweetened apricot or strawberry jam
- 2 fresh egg white

1. Put the cream cheese into the bowl and stir in the jam.

2. Combine well.

3. Create small slits in the center of each slice of bread, then fill it with the cream cheese and jam mixture.

4. In a bowl, whisk together the egg, fresh egg white, milk, and vanilla extract.

5. Add a dash of apple pie spice and whisk until foamy.

6. Place a nonstick skillet over medium low flame.

7. Carefully dip each slice of bread into the fresh egg mixture, then place on the hot skillet. Easy cook each slice for about 1-5 minutes per side, or until golden brown.

8. Transfer all the pieces onto a platter lined with heavy duty kitchen paper towels.

9. Serve warm.

Tostadas With Black Bean And Salmon

Ingredients

- Canola oil easily cooking spray

- 2 2 10 -ounce can black beans, drained and rinsed

- 4 tablespoons chopped cilantro

- 6 tablespoons reduced-fat sour cream

- 4 scallions, chopped

- 4 tablespoons prepared salsa

- Lime wedges

- 16 pieces 6-inch corn tortillas

- 10-15-ounce can skinless, boneless wild Alaskan salmon, liquid drained

- 4 tablespoons minced pickled jalapeños

133

- 4 tablespoons pickling juice from the pickled jalapeno jar, divided

- 2 medium avocado, diced

- 4 cups shredded cabbage or coleslaw mix

Easy make

1. Put oven racks in the lower and upper third positions.

2. Prepare oven temperature to 350 F. Spray both sides of each tortilla lightly with some easily cooking spray.

3. Arrange the tortilla on 4 cookie or baking sheets.

4. Bake tortilla in the oven, turning once for even cooking.

5. Bake until both sides are lightly browned, about 10 to 15 minutes.

6. Put avocado, jalapeno and salon in a bowl.

7. Toss to mix.

8. Get another bowl.

9. Put pickling juice, cilantro and cabbage.

10.   Mix and set aside.

11.   Put sour cream, scallions, salsa and black beans in a food processor.

12.   Pulse until mixture really really become smooth.

13.   Transfer the black bean mixture into a microwave-safe bowl.

14.   Heat on high for 1-5 minutes until hot.

15.	Alternatively, transfer into a saucepan and put over high heat until mixture is hot.

16.	Stir to just keep the bottom of the mixture from burning.

17.	Place one tortilla on a plate or chopping board.

18.	Spread some of the bean mixture over each tortilla.

19.	Top with some of the salmon mixture.

20.	Add some of the cabbage salad on top.

21.	Roll up or fold the tortilla in two. Serve with lime wedges.

Open-Face Tuna Salad

- 4 tablespoons extra-virgin olive oil

- 4 tablespoons chopped fresh parsley

- 4 green onions, sliced

- 2 10 -ounce can low-sodium tuna packed in water, drained

- 4 tablespoons freshly squeezed lemon juice

- Black pepper

- 1/2 cup fresh arugula

- 1/2 cup reduced-fat whipped cream cheese

- 4 slices multigrain bread

- 1/2 cup halved cherry tomatoes

137

Easy make

1. Combine lemon juice, green onion, pepper, parsley and oil in a bowl.

2. Put tuna in a separate bowl.

3. Pour about 1/2 of oil-juice mixture over the tune.

4. Reserve the remaining mixture.

5. Mix tuna and oil-juice mixture well.

6. Coat both sides of the bread lightly with the reserved oil-juice mixture.

7. Toast the bread until golden on both sides. Set aside.

8. Pour any remaining oil-juice mixture over the arugula.

9. Toss to mix. Spoon about 4 tablespoons cream cheese over each toast.

10.   Spread evenly over one side of the bread.

11.   Spoon half of the tuna mixture over each bread slice.

12.   Arrange half of the arugula then half of the cherry tomatoes over the tuna.

13.   Serve.

Salmon Salad & Pita

Ingredients:

4 tbsp. red onion (minced)

2 tbsp. lemon juice

8 tbsp. plain low-fat yogurt

½ cups salmon (canned)

8 pieces whole wheat pita bread

8 lettuce leaves

Ground black pepper to taste

A pinch of dill (dried or fresh)

4 tsp. capers (chopped or minced)

Directions:

1. Mix all the ingredients in a medium bowl.

2. Place 1 lettuce leaf and 2 cup of salmon salad into each pita bread.

3. Add the mixture before serving.

Dash Tuna Melt

Ingredients:

2 cup onion (chopped)

2 cup celery (chopped)

10 oz. canned white tuna (drained)

Salt and pepper to taste

8 oz. low-fat cheddar cheese (grated)

6 whole wheat English muffins

2 cup low-fat salad dressing (any brand)

Directions:

1. Pre-heat broiler to 150 F.

2. In a small bowl meanwhile, combine salad dressing, onion, celery and tuna.

3. Mix well.

4. Add salt and pepper

5. Toast the English muffins.

6. Put its split side-ups on a baking sheet and top each with 2 of tuna mixture.

7. Place the muffins into the broiler and heat for 10 to 15   minutes.

8. Top it with cheese and heat for another 5 to 10   minutes or until melt.

9. Remove the muffins from broiler and let it just cool for a minute.

Portobello Mushrooms With Florentine Sauce

Ingredients

- 4 large portobello mushrooms, stems removed
- Easily cooking spray
- 2 cup fresh baby spinach
- 4 large Eggland's Best fresh eggs
- 1/7 teaspoon salt
- 1/2 cup crumbled goat or feta cheese
- Minced fresh basil, optional
- 1/7 teaspoon garlic salt
- 1/7 teaspoon pepper
- 1 teaspoon olive oil
- 2 small onion, chopped

Directions

1. Preheat oven to 450 °. Spritz mushrooms with easily cooking spray; place in a 2 10 x2 0x2 -in. pan, stem side up.

2. Sprinkle with garlic salt and pepper.

3. Bake, uncovered, until tender, about 20 minutes.

4. Meanwhile, in a nonstick skillet, heat oil over medium-high heat; saute onion until tender.

5. Stir in spinach until wilted.

6. Whisk together fresh eggs and salt; add to skillet.

7. Easy cook and stir until fresh eggs are thickened and no liquid fresh egg remains; spoon onto mushrooms.

8. Sprinkle with cheese and, if desired, basil.

Cannellini Bean Hummus

Ingredients

- 1/2 teaspoon crushed red pepper flakes
- 4 tablespoons minced fresh parsley
- Pita breads, cut into wedges
- Assorted fresh vegetables
- 4 garlic cloves, peeled
- 2 can cannellini beans, rinsed and drained
- 1/2 cup tahini
- 6 tablespoons lemon juice
- 2 -1 teaspoons ground cumin
- 1/2 teaspoon salt

Directions

1. Place garlic in a food processor; cover and process until minced.

2. Add the beans, tahini, lemon juice, cumin, salt and pepper flakes; cover and process until smooth.

3. Transfer to a small bowl; stir in parsley.

4. Refrigerate until serving.

5. Serve with pita wedges and assorted fresh vegetables.

Honey-Wheat Dash Bread

Ingredients:

- 6 tablespoons of flaxseed;

- 6 tablespoons of poppy seeds;

- 6 tablespoons of sesame seeds;

- ¼ cup of flaxseed meal;

- ¼ cup of soy flour;

- 5-10 tablespoons of yeast;

- 10 cups of unbleached white flour; and

- A cup of dry rolled oats.

- 2 cup of applesauce (unsweetened);

- 2 tablespoon of sea salt;

- 2 cup honey;

- 1 cup of olive oil;

- 6 cups of water;

- 6 cups of whole wheat flour;

Instructions:

1. Mix together the water and dry rolled oats.
2. Microwave the mixture to about 250 degrees Fahrenheit for 1-5 minute before removing.
3. In a separate bowl, mix together the salt, yeast, seeds, flaxseed meal, soy flour and whole-wheat flour.
4. When done, throw in the oil, honey, and applesauce and continue mixing again until well combined.

5. Throw in the hot rolled oats that you microwave earlier and continue mixing for another 5-10 minutes while gradually adding in the white flour until your dough turns elastic and smooth.
6. Put a cover on the bowl and let the dough rise for about 2-2 ½ hours to twice its original size.
7. Once raised, divide the dough into 5-10 pieces, from which you'll create the loaves of your honey wheat bread.
8. Spray oil or easily cooking spray on loaf pans on which you'll bake the bread loaves to just keep the bread from sticking to them as you bake.
9. After putting the loaves on the loaf pans, let it rise for another 2-2 ½ hours.
10. After the final rise, bake the loaves for 45 to 50 minutes at 350 degrees Fahrenheit or just until the loaves

really become golden in color at the top.

11.   Let the loaves just cool outside the oven when done before enjoying.

Dashing Omelet

Ingredients:

- 4 cups of fresh spinach, torn;

- 4 tablespoons of fresh parsley;

- 16 eggs, fresh; and

- Easily cooking spray (non-stick).

- 1/7 teaspoon of cayenne pepper;

- 2 cup of low fat cheddar cheese, shredded;

- 1/7 teaspoon of salt;

Easily cooking

For the red pepper relish:

- 2 tablespoon of cider vinegar; and
- 1/2   cup red pepper, chopped.
- 1 teaspoon black pepper;
- 4 tablespoons green onion, chopped finely;

Instructions:

1. Coat your non- stick skillet with easily cooking spray then heat the thing on your stove.
2. Prepare the red pepper relish by mixing all the red pepper relish ingredients.
3. In another bowl, mix together the chives, salt, cayenne pepper, and eggs.
4. Use a wire whisk to have an easier time beating the ingredients together.
5. Pour the fresh egg mixture on your hot skillet.

6. Gently stir the mixture in the skillet until you see the center really become cooked, even if the sides are still liquid.
7. At this point, continue easily cooking for a minute more or until the whole mixture has set.
8. Sprinkle the shredded cheese on top before topping the omelet with the red pepper relish mixture.
9. Fold the omelet, remove from the skillet and enjoy!

Peanut Butter And Banana Smoothie

Ingredients

2 Tablespoon unsalted natural peanut

2 Teaspoon unsweetened cocoa powder (Option)

8 Ice cubes

2 Cup banana, peeled and sliced

2 Cup milk (skimmed)

2 Teaspoon vanilla extract (pure)

Preparation

1.   Place all your ingredients into your blender

2.   Process until the mixture is smooth

3.   Serve immediately

Parfait In Blue, White, And Red

2 Cup Blueberries

8 Teaspoons honey

4 Cups Greek yogurt (plain, non-fat)

2 Cup cherries pitted and halved

2 Cup raspberries

Preparation

1.　　　Layer 1　cup of cherries, 1-5 tablespoons of yogurt, 1　cup of blueberries, 1-5　tablespoons of yogurt 1　cup of raspberries and 4 tablespoons of yogurt in each of the 8 glasses.

2.   Drizzle each of the 8   parfaits
with 2 teaspoon of honey

Goat Cheese, Cherry Tomatoes, And Asparagus Pasta

- 1/2 cup fresh basil 2 tbsp garlic (minced)

- 1/7 tsp black pepper 4 oz. (60 g) soft goat cheese

- 1/2 lb (2 10 0 g) whole-wheat penne pasta

- 1 cup asparagus (chopped)

- 2 tbsp water

- 1 cup cherry tomatoes (halved)

Directions:

1. Place the pasta in a pot of boiling water and easy cook 20 to 25 minutes, following the package instructions.

2. Transfer to a colander to drain.

3. Meanwhile, place the asparagus and water in a microwave-safe bowl and heat the asparagus on HIGH until it is just softened, about 1-5 minutes.

4. In a bowl, place together the cherry tomatoes, garlic, basil and pepper.

5. Add the pasta, asparagus, and goat cheese and mix to coat.

6. Chill for at least 55 to 60 minutes to cool.

7. Place the pasta in a serving plate, decorate with fresh basil leaves and enjoy.

Sesame Tuna Salad

- 4 (10 -6 oz.) cans water-packed chunk light tuna (drained)
- 2 cup sugar snap peas or snow peas (sliced)
- 4 scallions (sliced)
- 12 cups Napa cabbage (thinly sliced)
- 8 radishes (sliced)
- 1/2 cup fresh cilantro leaves
- 2 tbsp sesame seeds
- Freshly ground pepper to taste
- 1/2 cup rice vinegar or lemon juice
- 6 tbsp canola oil
- 4 tbsp reduced-sodium soy sauce
- 2 tbsp toasted sesame oil

- 2 1 tsp sugar

- 2 1 tsp fresh ginger (minced)

Preparation:

1. In a small bowl, mix together the soy sauce, vinegar sesame oil, canola oil, ginger and sugar.

2. Combine tuna, scallions and peas in a medium bowl and spoon 1-5 tablespoons of dressing over the mixture.

3. Toss to coat.

4. Divide and place the sliced cabbage in 8 serving plates. Top with tuna mixture and sprinkle with sesame seeds, radishes and cilantro.

5. Drizzle the remaining dressing over the dish, season with pepper and enjoy!

Pancakes with Almond Flour

INGREDIENTS

- 2 cup almond flour
- 2 fresh egg
- 2 tsp vanilla extract
- 1 tsp baking soda
- salt
- ¼ cup milk
- sliced fruits

1. Preheat griddle to 350F

2. In a bowl whisk together baking soda, salt, almond flour, eggs, milk and vanilla extract

3. Pour the mixture on the griddle and easy cook each pancake for 5 to 10 minutes per side

4. Remove and serve with fruit and maple syrup on top

Blueberry Pancakes

- 2 cup tapioca flour
- *2 fresh egg*
- 1 cup avocado oil
- 4 tablespoons cane sugar
- 4 tsp almond extract
- 2 tsp baking powder
- 2 cups buckwheat flour
- 2 cups water
- 1 tsp baking soda
- 1 tsp salt
- 2 cups blueberry

- juice from 2 lemons

1. Easy make the pancakes mixture the night before easily cooking

2. In a bowl mix buckwheat flour, lemon juice, water and stir

3. In the morning add the rest of the ingredients in the mixture

4. In a skillet pour the pancakes mixture and easy cook 5 to 10 minutes per side

Blueberry Waffles

Ingredients:

- 6 tbsp. unsalted butter, melted
- 6 tbsp. nonfat plain Greek yogurt
- 2 1 c. 2 % milk
- 4 tsp. vanilla extract
- 8 ounces blueberries
- Nonstick easily cooking spray
- 1 c. maple almond butter
- 4 c. whole wheat flour
- 2 tbsp. baking powder
- 2 tsp. ground cinnamon

- 4 tbsp. sugar

- 4 large fresh eggs

Directions:

1. Preheat waffle iron.

2. Mix the flour, baking powder, cinnamon, plus sugar in a large bowl.

3. Mix the eggs, melted butter, yogurt, milk, and vanilla in a small bowl.

4. Combine well.

5. Put the wet fixing to the dry mix and whisk until well combined.

6. Do not over whisk; it's okay if the mixture has some lumps.

7. Fold in the blueberries.

8. Oiled the waffle iron with easily cooking spray, then easy cook 1/2   c. of the

batter until the waffles are lightly browned and slightly crisp.

9. Repeat with the rest of the batter.

10.   Place 4 waffles in each of 5-10 storage containers.

11.   Store the almond butter in 5-10 condiment cups.

12.   To serve, top each warm waffle with 2 tbsp.

13.   of maple almond butter.

Apple Pancakes

Ingredients:

- 2 c. 2 % milk
- 4 large fresh eggs
- 2 medium Gala apple, diced
- 4 tbsp. maple syrup
- 2 /8 c. chopped walnuts
- 1/2   c. extra-virgin olive oil, divided
- 2 c. whole wheat flour
- 4 tsp. baking powder
- 2 tsp. baking soda
- 2 tsp. ground cinnamon

Directions:

1. Set aside 2 tsp. of oil to use for greasing a griddle or skillet.

2. In a large bowl, stir the flour, baking powder, baking soda, cinnamon, milk, eggs, apple, and the remaining oil.

3. Warm griddle or skillet on medium-high heat and coat with the reserved oil. Working in batches, pour in about 1/2 c. of the batter for each pancake.

4. Easy cook until browned on both sides.

5. Place 5-10 pancakes into each of 5-10 medium storage containers and the maple syrup in 5-10 small containers.

6. Put each serving with 2 tbsp. of walnuts and drizzle with 1 tbsp. of maple syrup.

www.ingramcontent.com/pod-product-compliance
Lightning Source LLC
Chambersburg PA
CBHW060502030426
42337CB00015B/1695